CHAIR PILATES FOR SENIORS OVER 60

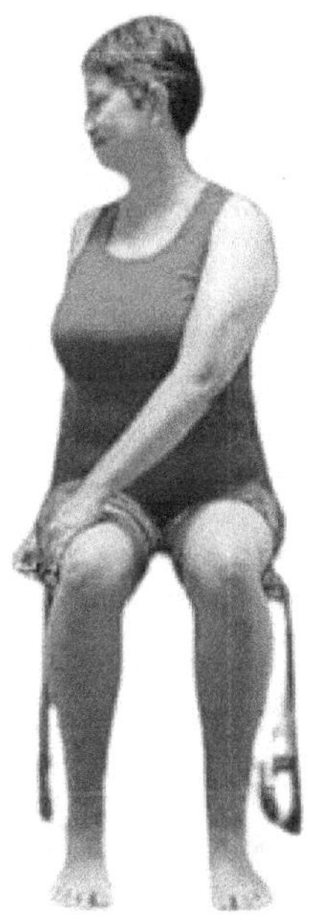

The Easy Step By Step Guide For Older People To Improve Physical Strength, Flexibility And Posture, Enhance Mental Awareness And Reshape Your Body Movements

Silvanus Bekee

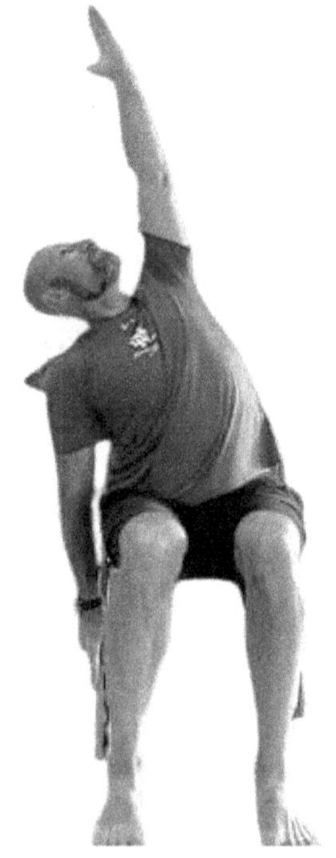

Table of Contents

INTRODUCTION

Imagine a world where the golden years are filled with vitality, flexibility, and a zest for life. Meet Jane, a spirited 68-year-old who discovered the transformative power of Chair Pilates for seniors over 60. Struggling with stiffness and limited mobility, she hesitantly embraced this accessible fitness guide, and what unfolded was nothing short of a rejuvenation journey.

As Jane committed to the gentle yet effective exercises outlined in this guide, a remarkable metamorphosis occurred. The chair became her gateway to renewed strength, balance, and improved posture. She reveled in the liberating feeling of regaining control over her body, effortlessly moving through exercises tailored to her comfort and ability. Chair Pilates became her daily ritual, a source of joy and empowerment that transcended the physical, seeping into the realms of mental clarity and emotional well-being. Now, imagine unlocking this transformative experience for yourself or your loved ones through our guide to chair Pilates for seniors over 60. This comprehensive resource is not just a collection of exercises; it's a roadmap to reclaiming vitality and embracing a more active lifestyle, all from the comfort of a chair. We understand the unique needs and considerations of seniors, offering a tailored approach to exercise that prioritizes safety and effectiveness.

Why chair Pilates? It's the gentle yet powerful gateway to enhanced strength, improved balance, and a renewed sense of well-being. In the pages that follow, we demystify the practice, providing step-by-step instructions, accompanied by vivid illustrations, making it accessible for everyone, regardless of fitness level.

As you delve into this guide, you'll discover how chair Pilates goes beyond physical benefits, addressing mental clarity and emotional resilience. Join us on this inspiring journey, where age becomes just a number, and every seated movement becomes a step towards a healthier, more vibrant life. Embrace the transformative power of chair Pilates – your body, mind, and spirit will thank you.

CHAPTER 1

Understanding Chair Pilates

Understanding chair Pilates involves recognizing it as a modified form of traditional Pilates, tailored specifically for individuals who may face challenges with mobility or prefer a seated workout. This low-impact exercise method combines elements of strength training, flexibility, and mindfulness, making it accessible for seniors or those with physical limitations.

The essence of chair Pilates lies in adapting classic Pilates exercises to a seated position, utilizing the chair as a stable base for various movements. This approach ensures that participants can engage in a full-body workout without putting excessive strain on joints or muscles. The exercises often focus on core strength, flexibility, and balance, addressing key aspects of overall well-being.

Moreover, understanding chair Pilates involves appreciating its versatility. It caters to different fitness levels, allowing individuals to progress at their own pace. The incorporation of controlled breathing further enhances the mind-body connection, promoting relaxation and stress reduction.

Ultimately, chair Pilates stands as an inclusive fitness option, offering a pathway to improved physical health and vitality, irrespective of age or physical condition. Whether used as a primary exercise routine or as a complementary practice, grasping the fundamentals of chair Pilates opens the door to a more accessible and enjoyable approach to fitness and well-being.

Safety Precautions And Guidelines

1. Consult with a Healthcare Professional: Before starting any chair Pilates program, consult with your healthcare provider to ensure it's safe given your individual health conditions.

2. Adapt to Your Comfort Level: Modify exercises based on your comfort level and physical abilities. It's essential to avoid pushing yourself too hard, especially if you're a beginner or dealing with pre-existing conditions.

3. Stable Seating: Use a stable and sturdy chair with a backrest. Ensure it is placed on a non-slip surface to prevent any accidental slips or falls during exercises.

4. Proper Body Alignment: Maintain proper body alignment throughout exercises. Pay attention to your posture, keeping your back straight and shoulders relaxed to avoid unnecessary strain.

5. Warm-Up and Cool Down: Begin each session with a gentle warm-up to prepare your muscles and joints. Similarly, incorporate a cool-down routine to gradually ease out of the exercises and reduce the risk of stiffness.

6. Breath Awareness: Focus on mindful breathing during exercises. Inhale deeply through your nose, and exhale slowly through your mouth. This not only enhances the effectiveness of the exercises but also promotes relaxation.

7. Stay Hydrated: Hydration is key. Keep water within reach and take regular sips throughout your session to prevent dehydration, especially if your chair Pilates routine is of moderate to high intensity.

8. Avoid Overexertion: Listen to your body and avoid overexertion. If you experience pain, discomfort, or dizziness, stop the exercise immediately and seek guidance from a healthcare professional.

9. Regular Breaks: Take short breaks between exercises to prevent fatigue and allow your body to recover. This is particularly important for seniors to avoid overexertion.

10. Clear Space: Ensure you have a clear and clutter-free space around your chair to avoid any tripping hazards. This is crucial for maintaining a safe environment during your chair Pilates sessions.

Core Benefits Of Chair Pilates For Seniors Over 60

1. Improved Core Strength: Chair Pilates targets core muscles, enhancing strength in the abdomen, lower back, and pelvic region. This contributes to better stability and balance, crucial for seniors to maintain an active lifestyle.

2. Enhanced Flexibility: The gentle stretching and range of motion exercises in chair Pilates help seniors improve flexibility in their joints and muscles, reducing stiffness and promoting ease of movement.

3. Better Posture: By focusing on proper body alignment and engaging core muscles, chair Pilates helps seniors develop and maintain good posture. Improved posture contributes to overall well-being and reduces the risk of musculoskeletal issues.

4. Increased Circulation: Chair Pilates incorporates controlled breathing, which, coupled with movement, promotes better blood circulation. Improved circulation can have positive effects on cardiovascular health and overall vitality.

5. Joint Mobility: The fluid movements in chair Pilates contribute to increased joint mobility. This is particularly beneficial for seniors, as it aids in preventing stiffness and supports overall joint health.

6. Stress Reduction: Mindful breathing and the rhythmic nature of chair Pilates exercises contribute to stress reduction. This practice provides seniors with a calming and meditative experience, fostering mental well-being.

7. Better Balance: Chair Pilates emphasizes stability and balance, crucial aspects for seniors to prevent falls. The targeted exercises enhance proprioception, allowing seniors to move confidently and reduce the risk of accidents.

8. Muscle Endurance: Regular participation in chair Pilates builds muscle endurance, allowing seniors to perform daily activities with greater ease and reduced fatigue. This is particularly beneficial for maintaining independence in daily life.

9. Pain Management: Chair Pilates can assist in managing chronic pain by promoting gentle movements that alleviate tension in muscles and joints. Seniors may experience relief from conditions such as arthritis or back pain.

10. Social Connection: Participating in chair Pilates classes or groups provides seniors with a social outlet. The shared experience fosters a sense of community and support, positively impacting mental and emotional well-being.

Warm Up Exercises

1. Neck Rotation:

- Starting Position:

Seated comfortably with feet flat on the floor and hands resting on thighs.

- Steps:

Gently turn your head to the right, hold for a moment, then rotate it to the left. Repeat, maintaining a slow and controlled pace.

- Repetition:

8-10 times each side.

- Purpose:

This exercise promotes neck flexibility, reducing tension and improving range of motion.

2. Shoulder Rolls:

- Starting Position:

Seated with a straight back and relaxed shoulders.

- Steps:

Lift shoulders towards the ears, roll them back in a circular motion, and then down. Reverse the direction after a few rolls.

- Repetition:

10-12 rolls in each direction.

- Purpose:

Shoulder rolls help release tension, improve posture, and enhance overall shoulder mobility.

3. Seated Marching:

- Starting Position:

Seated with feet hip-width apart and hands resting on the sides of the chair.

- Steps:

Lift one knee towards the chest, then lower it while lifting the other knee. Continue alternating in a controlled, rhythmic manner.

- Repetition:

20-25 marches.

- Purpose:

This exercise warms up the hip flexors, engages the core, and promotes circulation in the lower body.

4. Spinal Twist:

- Starting Position:

Seated with feet flat, hands on opposite sides of the chair.

- Steps:

Inhale and lengthen your spine, exhale and twist your torso to the right, using the chair for support. Hold briefly, then switch to the left side.

- Repetition:

6-8 twists on each side.

- Purpose:

The spinal twist mobilizes the spine, stretches the back muscles, and enhances overall spinal flexibility.

5. Ankle Circles:

- Starting Position:

Seated with feet flat on the floor.

- Steps:

Lift one foot slightly off the floor and rotate the ankle clockwise, then counter-clockwise. Repeat with the other foot.

- Repetition:

8-10 circles in each direction for each foot.

- Purpose:

Ankle circles improve ankle flexibility, reduce stiffness, and help with overall lower limb mobility.

CHAPTER 2

CHAIR PILATES

1. Seated Leg Lifts:

- Starting Position:

Sit upright with feet flat on the floor.

- Steps:

Lift one leg straight out, hold briefly, then lower it. Repeat with the other leg.

- Repetition:

12-15 lifts for each leg.

- Purpose:

Strengthens the quadriceps and improves overall leg strength and flexibility.

2. Chair Squats:

- Starting Position:

Sit at the edge of the chair with feet hip-width apart.

- Steps:

Stand up, extending hips forward, then lower back into the chair.

- Repetition:

10-12 squats.

- Purpose:

Targets the muscles in the lower body, enhancing strength and stability.

3. Seated Torso Twist:

- Starting Position:

Sit tall with hands on the sides of the chair.

- Steps:

Twist your torso to the right, then to the left, keeping the movement controlled.

- Repetition:

8-10 twists on each side.

- Purpose:

Engages the obliques, improving core strength and spinal mobility.

4. Arm Circles:

- Starting Position:

Sit comfortably with arms extended to the sides.

- Steps:

Make small circles with your arms, first clockwise, then counter-clockwise.

- Repetition:

12-15 circles in each direction.

- Purpose:

Enhances shoulder flexibility and strengthens the muscles in the arms.

5. Seated Marching with Arm Reach:

- Starting Position:

Sit with feet flat, arms by your sides.

- Steps:

Lift one knee towards your chest while reaching the opposite arm forward. Alternate sides.

- Repetition:

15-20 marches.

- Purpose:

Integrates leg and arm movements, promoting coordination and engaging the core.

6. Knee Extensions:

- Starting Position:

Seated with feet flat, extend one leg straight in front of you.

- Steps:

Hold the extended position for a moment, then lower the leg. Repeat with the other leg.

- Repetition:

10-12 extensions per leg.

- Purpose:

Targets the muscles in the thighs and improves overall leg strength.

7. Pelvic Tilts:

- Starting Position:

Sit tall with hands on your hips.

- Steps:

Tilt your pelvis forward and backward in a controlled manner.

- Repetition:

15-20 tilts.

- Purpose:

Strengthens the muscles around the pelvis, promoting better posture and core stability.

8. Seated Side Leg Lifts:

- Starting Position:

Sit with legs together, hands on the sides of the chair.

- Steps:

Lift one leg to the side, then lower it. Repeat with the other leg.

- Repetition:

12-15 lifts for each leg.

- Purpose:

Targets the outer thighs and hips, enhancing hip strength and stability.

9. Chair Dips:

- Starting Position:

Sit at the edge of the chair with hands gripping the seat.

- Steps:

Slide off the chair, bending your elbows as you lower your body, then push back up.

- Repetition:

10-12 dips.

- Purpose:

Works the triceps and strengthens the muscles in the upper body.

10. Seated Heel Raises:

- Starting Position:

Sit with feet flat on the floor.

- Steps:

Lift your heels off the ground, then lower them back down.

- Repetition: 15-20 heel raises.

- Purpose:

Targets the calf muscles, improving ankle mobility and lower leg strength.

11. Seated Toe Taps:

- Starting Position:

Sit with feet flat on the floor.

- Steps:

Tap one foot on the floor in front of you, then switch to the other foot.

- Repetition:

20-25 taps per foot.

- Purpose:

Activates the muscles in the lower legs and promotes ankle flexibility.

12. Seated Chest Opener:

- Starting Position:

Sit tall with hands clasped behind your back.

- Steps:

Open your chest by squeezing your shoulder blades together, then release.

- Repetition:

12-15 chest openings.

- Purpose:

Improves posture and stretches the chest muscles.

13. Seated Knee Circles:

- Starting Position:

Sit with knees bent and feet flat on the floor.

- Steps:

Circle your knees in a clockwise, then counter-clockwise motion.

- Repetition:

10-12 circles in each direction.

- Purpose:

Enhances mobility in the knee joints and promotes circulation.

14. Seated Bicep Curls:

- Starting Position:

Sit with a straight back, holding a light weight in each hand.

- Steps:

Curl the weights towards your shoulders, then lower them back down.

- Repetition:

12-15 curls.

- Purpose:

Strengthens the biceps and improves arm strength.

15. Seated Side Bend:

- Starting Position:

Sit tall with hands on your hips.

- Steps:

Gently lean to one side, feeling a stretch along the opposite side of your torso. Return to the center and repeat on the other side.

- Repetition:

8-10 bends on each side.

- Purpose:

Stretches and strengthens the muscles along the sides of the torso.

16. Seated Wrist Circles:

- Starting Position:

Sit with hands resting on your thighs.

- Steps:

Circle your wrists clockwise, then counter-clockwise.

- Repetition:

10-12 circles in each direction.

- Purpose:

Promotes wrist flexibility and helps alleviate tension.

17. Seated Lateral Leg Raises:

- Starting Position:

Sit with feet together, hands on the sides of the chair.

- Steps:

Lift one leg to the side, then lower it. Repeat with the other leg.

- Repetition:

12-15 raises for each leg.

- Purpose:

Targets the outer thighs and hip muscles, enhancing overall hip strength.

18. Seated Ankle Flex and Point:

- Starting Position:

Sit with feet flat on the floor.

- Steps:

Flex your ankles by pointing toes upward, then point them downward.

- Repetition:

15-20 flex and point movements.

- Purpose:

Improves ankle mobility and stretches the muscles in the lower legs.

19. Seated Overhead Reach:

- Starting Position:

Sit with a straight back, arms by your sides.

- Steps:

Inhale and reach your arms overhead, lengthening your spine.

- Repetition:

10-12 overhead reaches.

- Purpose:

Stretches the spine, shoulders, and promotes improved upper body flexibility.

20. Seated Clamshells:

- Starting Position:

Sit with knees bent, feet flat on the floor.

- Steps:

Open and close your knees, engaging the outer hip muscles.

- Repetition:

12-15 clamshells.

- Purpose:

Strengthens the muscles around the hips, supporting hip joint stability.

21. Seated Calf Raises:

- Starting Position:

Sit with feet flat on the floor.

- Steps:

Lift your heels off the ground, raising your heels as high as comfortable.

- Repetition:

15-20 calf raises.

- Purpose:

Targets the calf muscles, improving lower leg strength and ankle stability.

22. Seated Forward Bend:

- Starting Position:

Sit tall with legs extended in front of you.

- Steps:

Hinge at the hips and reach forward towards your toes, keeping your back straight.

- Repetition:

Hold for 15-20 seconds, repeating 2-3 times.

- Purpose:

Stretches the hamstrings and promotes flexibility in the lower back.

23. Seated Arm Pulses:

- Starting Position:

Sit with a straight back, arms extended straight in front.

- Steps:

Pulse your arms up and down in a small, controlled movement.

- Repetition:

15-20 pulses.

- Purpose:

Activates the muscles in the arms and shoulders, promoting upper body strength.

24. Seated Hip Flexor Stretch:

- Starting Position:

Sit at the edge of the chair, one ankle crossed over the opposite knee.

- Steps:

Gently press down on the crossed knee, feeling a stretch in the hip.

- Repetition:

Hold for 15-20 seconds on each side, repeating 2-3 times.

- Purpose:

Stretches and releases tension in the hip flexors.

25. Seated Side Leg Circles:

- Starting Position:

Sit with legs extended, hands on the sides of the chair.

- Steps:

Lift one leg and make circular motions with your foot.

- Repetition:

8-10 circles in each direction for each leg.

- Purpose:

Improves hip joint mobility and strengthens the muscles around the thighs.

26. Seated Side Leg Swings:

- Starting Position:

Sit with legs extended, hands on the sides of the chair.

- Steps:

Swing one leg out to the side and back in a controlled manner. Repeat with the other leg.

- Repetition:

12-15 swings for each leg.

- Purpose:

Enhances hip flexibility and engages the outer thigh muscles.

27. Seated Abdominal Crunches:

- Starting Position:

Sit tall with hands behind your head.

- Steps:

Engage your core and lean back slightly, then return to the upright position.

- Repetition:

15-20 crunches.

- Purpose:

Targets the abdominal muscles, promoting core strength.

28. Seated Inner Thigh Squeezes:

- Starting Position:

Sit with a straight back and a small ball between your knees.

- Steps:

Squeeze the ball with your inner thighs, then release.

- Repetition:

12-15 squeezes.

- Purpose:

Strengthens the inner thigh muscles, improving overall leg stability.

29. Seated Side Reach:

- Starting Position:

Sit with a straight back, arms by your sides.

- Steps:

Reach one arm overhead to the opposite side, feeling a stretch along your torso. Repeat on the other side.

- Repetition:

8-10 reaches on each side.

- Purpose:

Stretches the side body and improves lateral flexibility.

30. Seated Leg Crosses:

- Starting Position:

Sit with legs extended, cross one leg over the other.

- Steps:

Hold the crossed position, feeling a stretch in the outer hip. Repeat with the other leg.

- Repetition:

Hold for 15-20 seconds on each side, repeating 2-3 times.

- Purpose:

Stretches the outer hip muscles and promotes hip joint flexibility.

SPECIAL MOTIVATIONAL QUOTES

1. Age is Just a Number:

- Embrace the journey with chair Pilates as a testament that age is merely a number. Every movement is a step towards a healthier, more vibrant you, breaking free from societal expectations.

2. Celebrate Your Progress:

- Recognize and celebrate even the smallest victories. Whether it's improved flexibility, increased strength, or a boost in energy, each step forward is a triumph worth acknowledging.

3. Invest in Your Well-being:

- Chair Pilates isn't just exercise; it's an investment in your overall well-being. By dedicating time to your health, you're laying the foundation for a more active, fulfilling life, regardless of age.

4. Community Support:

- Joining a chair Pilates group or class opens the door to a supportive community. Shared experiences and encouragement create a positive environment, making the journey more enjoyable and motivating.

5. Feel the Joy of Movement:

- Let the joy of movement be your driving force. Chair Pilates isn't about perfection; it's about enjoying the process, reveling in the newfound vitality that each session brings. Your body will thank you with increased energy and a sense of accomplishment.

CONCLUSION

In the concluding chapters of the chair Pilates guide for seniors over 60, we find ourselves at the intersection of newfound vitality and holistic well-being. The journey through the exercises has been more than a physical endeavor; it has been a transformative exploration of what it means to age with grace, resilience, and a commitment to one's health.

Chair Pilates, tailored for seniors, is not just a series of movements; it is a philosophy that challenges stereotypes and proves that age is not a barrier to adopting a healthier lifestyle. The guide has unfolded a tapestry of exercises targeting core strength, flexibility, balance, and overall fitness. More than just a fitness routine, chair Pilates has become a vehicle for self-care, an investment in physical and mental well-being.

As seniors engaged in these exercises, they discovered the joy of movement, a rhythm that transcends the limitations often associated with aging. The stories of participants, like

Margaret's journey from stiffness to flexibility, echo the broader narrative of triumph over physical constraints. Chair Pilates has not only rejuvenated bodies but fostered a sense of community, proving that the shared pursuit of health knows no age boundaries.

The emphasis on safety throughout the guide underscores the importance of considering individual health conditions. Chair Pilates is designed to be inclusive, allowing participants to adapt exercises to their comfort levels, promoting a sense of empowerment and control over their fitness journey.

As we conclude this guide, it is not merely a farewell but an invitation to continue this empowering journey. Chair Pilates for seniors over 60 is a timeless companion, offering a pathway to enhanced strength, improved flexibility, and a renewed zest for life. The chair has become more than just a prop; it is a symbol of support, stability, and the endless possibilities that unfold when one commits to their well-being. May each movement in the chair Pilates guide be a step towards a healthier, more active, and fulfilling life for all its readers.

FITNESS

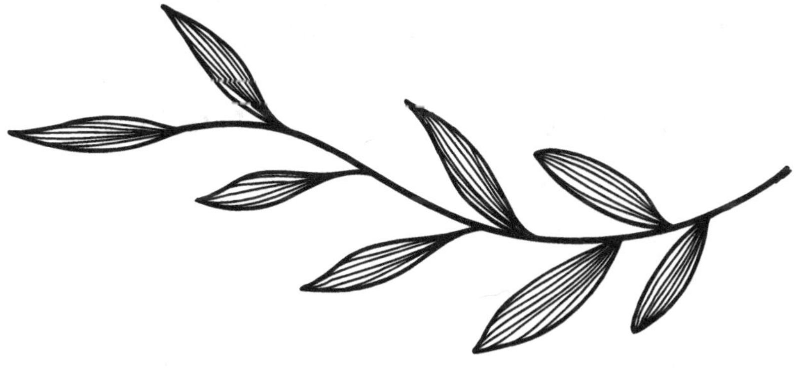

PLANNER

Fitness Planner

NAME: **DATE:**

BREAKFAST   **LUNCH**

DINNER   **SNACK**

EXERCISE   **SET**   **REP**   **NOTES**

Fitness Planner

NAME: **DATE:**

BREAKFAST

LUNCH

DINNER

SNACK

EXERCISE

EXERCISE	SET	REP	NOTES

Fitness Planner

NAME: **DATE:**

BREAKFAST

LUNCH

DINNER

SNACK

EXERCISE   SET   REP   NOTES

Fitness Planner

NAME: **DATE:**

BREAKFAST

LUNCH

DINNER

SNACK

EXERCISE

SET   REP   NOTES

Fitness Planner

NAME: **DATE:**

BREAKFAST   **LUNCH**

DINNER   **SNACK**

EXERCISE   **SET**   **REP**   **NOTES**

Fitness Planner

NAME: **DATE:**

BREAKFAST

LUNCH

DINNER

SNACK

EXERCISE

EXERCISE	SET	REP	NOTES

Fitness Planner

NAME: **DATE:**

BREAKFAST

LUNCH

DINNER

SNACK

EXERCISE	SET	REP	NOTES

Fitness Planner

NAME: **DATE:**

BREAKFAST

LUNCH

DINNER

SNACK

EXERCISE	SET	REP	NOTES

Fitness Planner

NAME: **DATE:**

BREAKFAST **LUNCH**

DINNER **SNACK**

EXERCISE	SET	REP	NOTES

Fitness
Planner

NAME: DATE:

BREAKFAST   LUNCH

DINNER   SNACK

EXERCISE   SET   REP   NOTES